# Lean Waist Warrior

# Workout Blast

By

# R.S Jacobs

www.leanwaistwarrior.com

Copyright © 2016

# Table of contents

# Disclaimer

We encourage all participants to eat a healthy, well balanced diet in conjunction with this workout plan, in order to ensure you achieve your desired goal. People with heart conditions or other physical related illnesses should endeavour to consult a physician before partaking in this workout routine. We do not make any claims or guarantees about the veracity of the result. Therefore, we do not accept any liabilities therein.

# Introduction

Our workout plan consists of carefully selected exercises, which are designed to be carried out as HIIT regime (**High Intensity Interval Training**).

HIIT is made up of short, sharp exercises at high intervals combined with rest periods in between (e.g. 15 squats in 30 seconds followed by 15 seconds of rest). The goal of HIIT is to elevate your heart rate to maximum levels, and then allow it to return to normal during your rest period.

We have three workout routines created by professional personal trainers. We advised that you start from the Bronze workout and then work your way up to the Gold workout Blast.

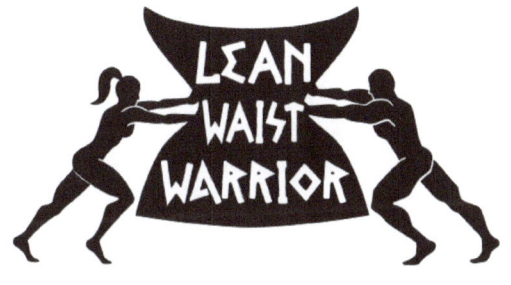

**Unleash your inner warrior**

# Lean Waist Warrior

## Bronze Workout

**For maximum results, do this workout 2-4 times a week.**

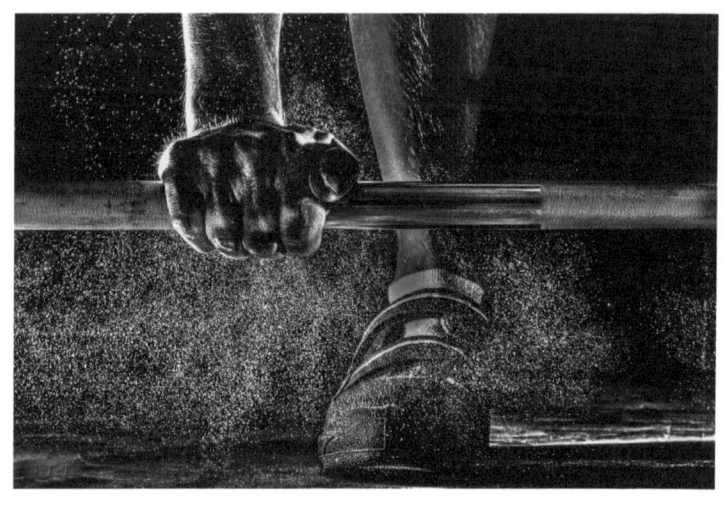

# Things you`ll need for LWW Workout

1. Water (1 Litre)

2. Towel

3. Weights (Kettlebells or Dumbbells x 2. Recommended weights: 5KG For Women and 10 KG For Men. Aim to increase the weights as you improve)

# Be ready for a fat melting workout BLAST

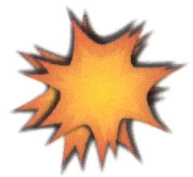

# Warm Up Circuit!

Arm Stretch (7 Secs on each arm)

Leg Stretch (7 Secs on each leg)

Toe Touches (10 Reps)

High Knees (10 Reps)

Jumping Jacks (10 Reps)

# The Body Blast Circuit

# (Non-stop Zone)

Burpees (30 sec)

Mountain Climbers (30 Sec)

Squat Jumps (30 Sec)

High Skater Hops (30 Sec)

Squat Taps (30 Sec)

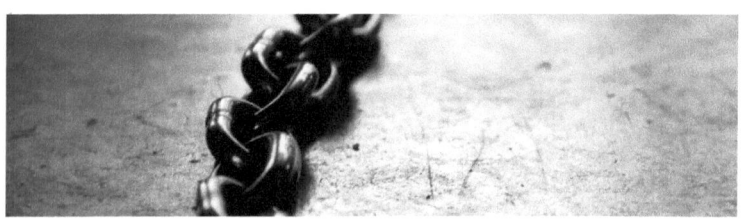

**Take a 30 second break and drink some water**

# The Toning Circuit

Dumbbell/Kettlebell Biceps Curls (30 reps)

Triceps Curls  (30 reps)

Ab Crunches (60 reps)

Squats (60 reps)

# Warm Down Circuit

Upper Leg Stretch

Hamstring Stretch

Bicep/Tricep Stretch

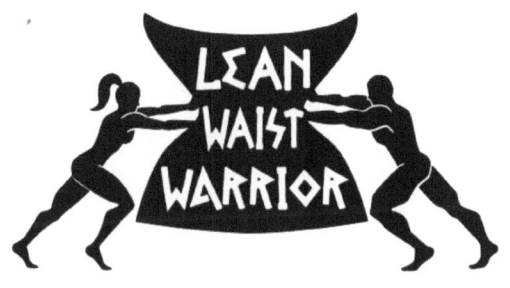

**Unleash your inner warrior**

# Lean Waist Warrior

## Silver Workout

**For maximum results, do this workout 2-4 times a week.**

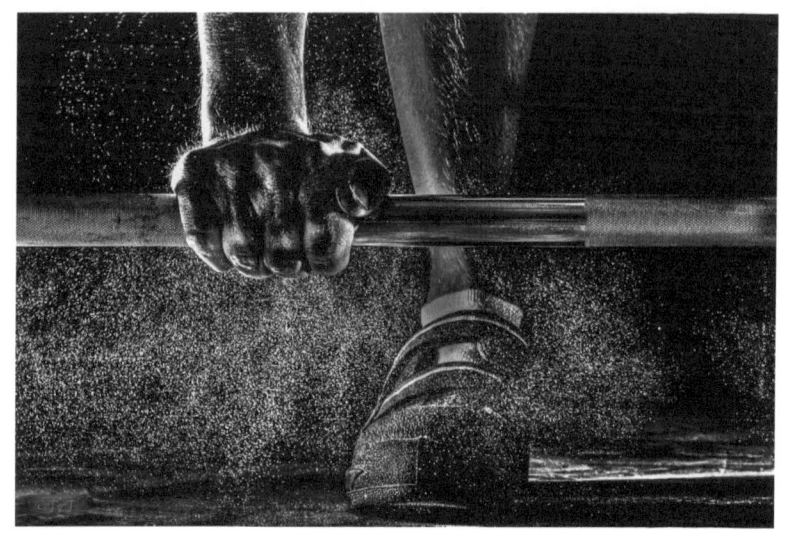

## Things you`ll need for LWW Workout

1. Water (1 Litre)

2. Towel

3. Weights (Kettlebells or Dumbbells x 2. Recommended weights: 5KG For Women and 10 KG For Men. Aim to increase the weights as you improve)

# Be ready for a fat melting workout BLAST

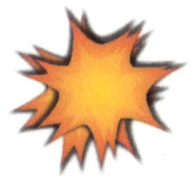

# Warm Up Circuit!

Arm Stretch (7 Secs on each arm)

Leg Stretch (7 Secs on each leg)

Toe Touches (10 Reps)

High Knees (10 Reps)

Jumping Jacks (10 Reps)

# The Body Blast Circuit

## (Non-stop Zone)

Push Ups (20 Reps)

Supersonic Fast Mountain Climbers (40 reps)

Skater Kicks (20 Reps)

Butt Kicks (40 Reps)

Cross Jacks (20 Reps)

Burpees (40 Reps)

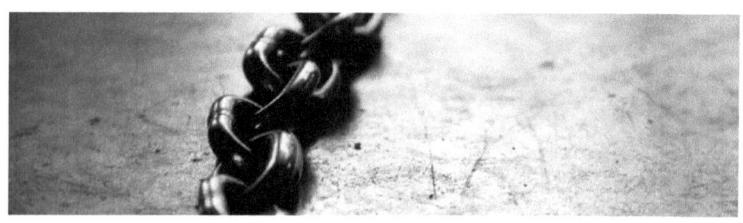

**Take a 30 second break and drink some water**

# The Toning Circuit

Dumbbell/Kettlebell Biceps Curls (30 reps)

Triceps Curls (30 reps)

Bicycle Crunches ( 30 reps)

Squats (60 reps)

Back Lunges & High Knees (30 Reps)

Russian Twists (30 Reps)

Planking (60 Seconds)

# Warm Down Circuit

Upper Leg Stretch

Hamstring Stretch

Bicep/Tricep Stretch

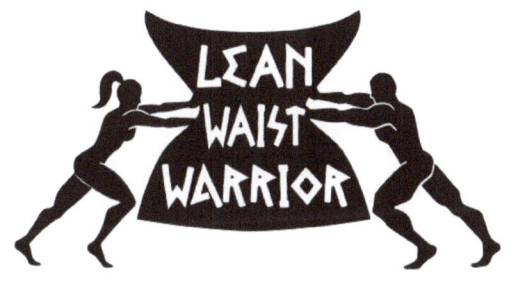

**Unleash your inner warrior**

# Lean Waist Warrior

## Gold Workout

**For maximum results, do this workout 2-4 times a week.**

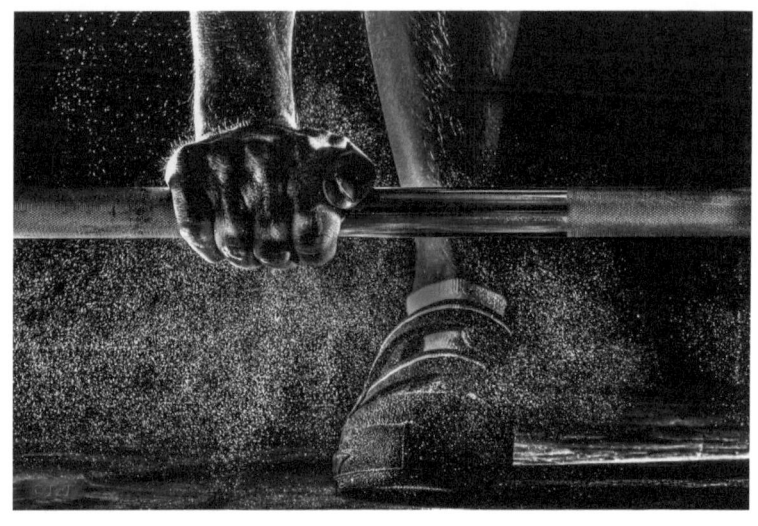

## Things you'll need for LWW Workout

1. Water (1 Litre)

2. Towel

3. Weights (Kettlebells or Dumbbells x 2. Recommended weights: 5KG For Women and 10 KG For Men. Aim to increase the weights as you improve)

# Be ready for a fat melting workout BLAST

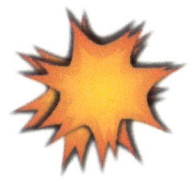

# Warm UP circuit!

Arm Stretch (7 Secs on each arm)

Leg Stretch (7 Secs on each leg)

Toe Touches (10 Reps)

High Knees (10 Reps)

Jumping Jacks (10 Reps)

Jogging On The Spot (20 Sec)

# The Body Blast Circuit

## (Non-stop Zone)

Push Ups (20 Reps)

Supersonic Fast Mountain Climbers (40 reps)

Skater Kicks (20 Reps)

Butt Kicks (40 Reps)

Cross Jacks (20 Reps)

Squat and Jab (40 Reps)

Burpees (20 Reps)

Kettlebell Swings (40 Reps)

Sit Ups (20 Reps)

Spider Push Ups (40 Reps)

**Take a 30 second break and drink some water**

# The Toning Circuit

Dumbbell/Kettlebell Biceps Curls (30 reps)

Triceps Curls (30 reps)

Farmer`s Deadlift (Kettlebell/Dumbbell in each hand) (30 Reps)

Bicycle Crunches ( 30 reps)

V-Sit Crunches (30 Reps)

Squats (60 reps)

Back Lunges & High Knees (30 Reps)

Russian Twists (30 Reps)

Planking (60 Seconds)

# Warm Down Circuit

Upper Leg Stretch

Hamstring Stretch

Bicep/Tricep Stretch

# STAY STRONG,
# WARRIOR!

# Other Books From Author

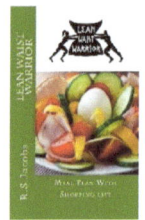

Lean Waist Warrior

Meal Plan with Shopping list


Available on Amazon

# The Writers
# Useful
# Compendium

A compendium of the highly successful '501
series' of publications providing short,
descriptive phrases, expressions and one liner's
to give your writing that extra punch … and
hopefully bring a smile to your face.

QUENTIN COPE

# COPYRIGHT & DISCLAIMER